Modern Social Policy